T0245444

CAMBRIDGE LIBRARY COLLECTION

Books of enduring scholarly value

History of Medicine

It is sobering to realise that as recently as the year in which On the Origin of Species was published, learned opinion was that diseases such as typhus and cholera were spread by a ‚Äòmiasma‚Äô, and suggestions that doctors should wash their hands before examining patients were greeted with mockery by the profession. The Cambridge Library Collection reissues milestone publications in the history of Western medicine as well as studies of other medical traditions. Its coverage ranges from Galen on anatomical procedures to Florence Nightingale‚Äôs common-sense advice to nurses, and includes early research into genetics and mental health, colonial reports on tropical diseases, documents on public health and military medicine, and publications on spa culture and medicinal plants.

A Letter on Sickness and Mortality in the West Indies

Sir Andrew Halliday (1782–1839) served as a surgeon in the Peninsular War, and then as a royal physician. In 1832 he was appointed Inspector of Hospitals in the West Indies until ill-health forced his return to Scotland. This 1839 pamphlet contains his recommendations to the Secretary of War, concerning the major losses suffered by the army in the West Indies due to illness. It was written in response to the Tulloch report presented to Parliament on the subject the previous year. This showed that the average death rate for soldiers there was almost six times higher that those in Britain, and in some islands considerably higher, due to dysentery, yellow fever and malaria. Halliday believed that many of these deaths were preventable, if medical advice was consulted on the siting of barracks, the daily regimes within them, and sanitation, and if doctors had the authority to implement changes.

Cambridge University Press has long been a pioneer in the reissuing of out-of-print titles from its own backlist, producing digital reprints of books that are still sought after by scholars and students but could not be reprinted economically using traditional technology. The Cambridge Library Collection extends this activity to a wider range of books which are still of importance to researchers and professionals, either for the source material they contain, or as landmarks in the history of their academic discipline.

Drawing from the world-renowned collections in the Cambridge University Library, and guided by the advice of experts in each subject area, Cambridge University Press is using state-of-the-art scanning machines in its own Printing House to capture the content of each book selected for inclusion. The files are processed to give a consistently clear, crisp image, and the books finished to the high quality standard for which the Press is recognised around the world. The latest print-on-demand technology ensures that the books will remain available indefinitely, and that orders for single or multiple copies can quickly be supplied.

The Cambridge Library Collection will bring back to life books of enduring scholarly value (including out-of-copyright works originally issued by other publishers) across a wide range of disciplines in the humanities and social sciences and in science and technology.

A Letter
on Sickness and
Mortality in the
West Indies

Being a Review of Captain Tulloch's
Statistical Report

SIR ANDREW HALLIDAY

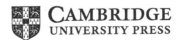

CAMBRIDGE
UNIVERSITY PRESS

CAMBRIDGE UNIVERSITY PRESS

Cambridge, New York, Melbourne, Madrid, Cape Town, Singapore,
São Paolo, Delhi, Dubai, Tokyo, Mexico City

Published in the United States of America by Cambridge University Press, New York

www.cambridge.org
Information on this title: www.cambridge.org/9781108023115

© in this compilation Cambridge University Press 2010

This edition first published 1839
This digitally printed version 2010

ISBN 978-1-108-02311-5 Paperback

ON

SICKNESS AND MORTALITY

IN THE

WEST INDIES.

A

LETTER

TO THE

RIGHT HON^BLE THE SECRETARY AT WAR,

ON

SICKNESS AND MORTALITY

IN THE

WEST INDIES;

BEING A REVIEW OF CAPTAIN TULLOCH'S
STATISTICAL REPORT.

BY

SIR ANDREW HALLIDAY, M.D., F.R.S.E.,

DEPUTY-INSPECTOR GENERAL OF ARMY HOSPITALS.

LONDON:

JOHN W. PARKER, WEST STRAND.

M.DCCC.XXXIX.

RIGHT HON. LORD VISCOUNT HOWICK,

SECRETARY AT WAR.

My Lord,

We are indebted to your Lordship's sound judgment and great humanity for the existence of a document which is confessedly of great importance, and calculated, more than any other that has ever yet been made public, to promote the best interests and general welfare of the British Army. I allude to the Statistical Report on the Sickness, Mortality, and Invaliding, among the Troops in the West Indies, as drawn up by Captain Tulloch, and presented to both Houses of Parliament during the last Session. In the introduction to that Report, Captain Tulloch informs us "That in October, 1835, your Lordship deemed it requisite that an inquiry should be instituted into the extent and causes of the sickness and mortality among the troops in the West Indies, with the view of founding thereon such measures as might appear likely to diminish the great loss of life annually experienced in these Colonies." There was no subject of inquiry, I venture to affirm, more worthy of your attention, as an officer of the Crown, nor any one

B

connected with your appointment as Secretary at War, that more urgently demanded a most thorough and searching investigation. Other Secretaries at War may have distinguished themselves by their knowledge of accounts, and the excellence of their official regulations— they may have earned praise for bringing into lucid order and regularity the whole system of our Military expenditure, and have framed good general orders for the strict discharge of the Soldier's duty; but, with the exception of your gallant and amiable predecessor — the TRUE SOLDIER, and the Soldier's TRUE FRIEND—Sir Henry Hardinge, I do not recollect any one, during the last forty years, who made the health or the happiness of the human being the subject of due consideration. Your Lordship, however, has now commenced this good work, and I trust you will cause it to be continued, until you are indeed able to found thereon such measures as may effectually diminish the great loss of life annually experienced in our West India and other Colonies.

It is to be most sincerely regretted that some officer in the medical department of the army was not deemed worthy of being recommended to your Lordship, as capable of discharging those duties which were assigned to Captain Tulloch. It has tended much to lower the department, already sufficiently low in the estimation of the public, and must prove most disheartening to every member of that department, to find a military subaltern earning promotion by the performance of a task that most especially belonged to the medical officer. Army medical men have now but few opportunities of earning either praise or promotion in or out of their department, and it shows but little zeal in their behalf, that they were passed over on this occasion. There are still many individuals connected with the Army Medical Department who are as able as Captain Tulloch, and not less willing to undertake the examination and condensation of the Medical and War-Office Returns; and some, I venture to assert, as conversant with Statistical details, and as capable of turning them to account, as the gallant captain, or any other military officer whatsoever. I readily allow, notwithstanding, that no man could have more ably fulfilled the duty which your Lordship intrusted to him, than Captain Tulloch has done. His Report is an interesting and invaluable document; and it is only because, as he states, that " it is principally confined to such points as can readily be solved by the test of facts and figures," and " to such matters *only* as can be made the subject of calculation," that I consider it of less importance than it might otherwise have been. A physician practically conversant with West India service, and at the same time a competent arithmetician, might have brought into view many causes of sickness and mortality, that can never be discovered by any accumulation of figures, and to discuss many matters which I firmly believe could never be made the subject of mere calculation.

There may be, and no doubt are, many medical officers more able than I am to discuss the several matters contained in this Report; yet, your Lordship is not quite ignorant of the anxious attention which I have given to the subject, and I feel more than an usual degree of pleasure in believing, as I certainly do, that it was owing to my letters from the West Indies in 1834, that the sickness and mortality among the troops in these colonies was forced upon the attention of men in authority, and that the subject was brought more immediately under your Lordship's notice. Every hour that I was allowed to remain in the West Indies was employed in investigating, upon the spot, the assigned or probable causes of the sickness and mortality that prevailed around me. I was then convinced, and still am, that many of the unknown, and most of the obvious and tangible causes of those diseases which are the principal source of mortality, may and can be removed by means fully within our power, and therefore I feel it a duty which I owe to myself, not less than to my fellow-creatures, to call your Lordship's attention to the observations I am now about to offer on Captain Tulloch's Statistical Report.

There was a time, my Lord, when we had on the active staff of the Army men who could and did investigate the causes and the consequences of the diseases which assailed the troops under their superintendence, and were not afraid to publish and support the opinions they had formed, or the treatment they considered necessary for the prevention, not less than the cure, of these diseases; and we had, too, military commanders that would listen to their opinions and seek their counsel; but, now alas, all *writing men* have apparently been excluded from the service. An Army Medical Officer must neither take a pen in his hand, nor open his mouth, except within the walls of the military-hospital.

There are still, I am proud to say, some men of talent, and certainly of great experience, among the medical

officers of the Army; but length of days, and the wear and
tear of unhealthy climates, do not generally improve the
intellect; and, though a more gentlemanly or better-
educated class of young men never existed than the junior
officers appointed by Sir James M'Grigor since the peace,
yet, what avails talent, if it is not to be appreciated,
or experience, or the strongest intellect, if not consulted;
or of what account is the best education, if it is not to be
encouraged and improved, with at least some chance of
reward? When I was in the West Indies, the medical
officers had entirely lost cast, and seemed scarcely acknow-
ledged: the commanding engineer had usurped all the
rights and privileges of the principal medical officer: the
idea of consulting the Inspector of Hospitals about the
locality or the construction of a barrack, how much
soever it might concern the health of the troops, would
have been considered as a condescension out of all
question, and even when the general hospital at Barbados was to be rebuilt after the hurricane of 1831, I
believe I am correct in stating that the Inspector-General
on the spot, Dr. Baxter, was never once asked where it
ought to be built, and far less how. The idea of a
DOCTOR presuming to offer an opinion as to the best construction of a barrack-room, or even of a sick-ward, was
evidently so much out of place, that when I ventured to
offer a suggestion during the progress of the building at
St. Ann's, I was laughed at.

No man living could show more anxiety for the welfare of the troops in the West Indies than my immediate
predecessor Dr. Bone, Deputy Inspector-General of Hospitals, nor was any health officer ever at greater pains to
inculcate such rules and regulations as his long experience

had proved to be of importance in preserving their health; but not one of his suggestions was attended to, and some of the most obvious of his recommendations for cleanliness and comfort, and for cooking their unwholesome messes, were never even adverted to by the military authorities.

The late good old Barrack-Master at Barbados, (Colonel Diggins) found out a process by which the most filthy and unfit ingredient then, and still, in use for stuffing the soldiers' palliasses, might be made a most clean and comfortable article of bedding, and twenty times more economical than that in use; and that it was so, was fully certified by Mr. Gunning, the Inspector-General of Hospitals at the time; but as it did not suit the Commissary-General to have any additional trouble imposed upon his department, and because it was recommended by a Doctor—no matter how much the poor soldier might suffer—no matter how often he might be driven to sleep upon the bare boards in the open galleries, or perhaps forced to the grog-shop to escape the myriads of bugs and vermin that were hatched in the stuffing of his palliass, and brought forth in swarms, ready to devour his body—no matter what number of punishments might take place for irregularities in a manner forced upon the unhappy sufferer, or what amount of sickness or mortality might ensue from the soldier finding it impossible to enjoy one moment of rest or of sound sleep—no matter as to all these considerations, the Commissariat routine could not be interfered with; the crude Indian corn husks continued in use up till 1836, and I fear still continue. In this case, my Lord, two lines of a General Order would not only have done away with the nuisance,

but have saved the lives of many brave men, and pre-
served the health of more.

I therefore do not hesitate to attribute very much of
the sickness that generally prevails, and not a little of
the mortality that follows, to that careless indifference
as to the common comforts and conveniences of the
soldier, which was so evident on West India service;
and to that total disregard of all measures of prevention, even when pointed out by the intelligent medical
officer.

Another source of the great mortality among our troops
in the West Indies, as connected with this branch of the
subject, deserves your serious attention, and certainly
calls for your Lordship's most decided interference. I
here allude to the too often injudicious manner in which
the soldiers are treated when attacked with sickness.
This arises from the bad organization of the medical
department itself. Men are now kept employed upon
the staff, when it is well known that both their bodily and
mental powers are greatly in abeyance, and who, instead
of being able to treat the sick soldiers themselves, or
to instruct others how to treat them, are scarcely able to
sign the numerous returns their clerks are called upon
to make out for the Medical Board Office; and young
men, almost immediately on their appointment to the
service, are hurried off to the West Indies; and however
well educated they may be, or "deep read in the theory
of physic," they can have but little practical experience in
the treatment of any class of diseases even in Europe,
and certainly none of those that are most common within
the tropics. And, as it very seldom happens that much
time is allowed to the most practised observer to study the

symptoms of West India diseases at the bed-side of the
patient, the physician must gain his knowledge of their
treatment by the frequency of their occurrence, and too
often acquire experience from the repeated failure of his
best endeavours to save his patient. Every inducement
therefore ought to be held out, not only to stimulate young
men of superior abilities to volunteer for this service, but
to encourage them to remain in the West Indies as long
as their health and constitutions can withstand the
climate. At present there is nothing to be gained by
any exertion, no stimulus whatever to acquire distinction.
However diligent and observing a man may be, or however much he may sacrifice his health or his ease to
cure the epidemic and endemial diseases of the colony in
which he may be stationed, the prospect of any reward,
or even of any praise, is now almost hopeless; nay, I
have actually known zeal procure censure. If a vacancy
occurs, the promotion, of late, has almost never been given
to the officer on the spot. A fresh man is sent out, who
again, in the course of what I may call his apprenticeship,
will lose many of the patients that his experienced predecessor would have saved. Disappointed of the reward
which he had hoped his zeal and his success might
have secured for him, the experienced officer now becomes
careless and indifferent, and is only anxious to get
removed from so dangerous a climate; while the newly
promoted (having nothing to excite his ambition), soon
becomes sick himself, or gets tired of the country, and
before he has acquired half the experience of the man he
has superseded, is employing his days and nights in
devising means to get away from it.

When a medical officer, by perseverance and a close

attention to the symptoms of disease, and the proper effects of remedies in the cases that are so frequent and so fatal in our West India Colonies, has acquired a knowledge of their character, and a success in treating them, I would then say, my Lord, that if the lives of our gallant soldiers are of the least account, the services of such a man are become invaluable—they are beyond all price, and ought undoubtedly to be secured either by some pecuniary reward, or professional promotion. It is not always, I grant, that a medical officer can be rewarded with promotion even in the West Indies; yet, when a vacancy does occur, it ought never to be given out of the command. Above all, your Lordship ought to contrive some means of keeping experienced officers in attendance upon the troops in the Colonies, by allowing them, after certain and fixed periods, to obtain local rank, with the pay and allowances of that rank, while they continue to remain on that service. The officers of the Ordnance, when sent to the West Indies, have what is called climate pay, a considerable addition to their ordinary pay. Why not then give something of the same sort to the medical staff officers, whose duties expose them to a thousand causes of sickness and mortality, that the military officer never has to encounter, and whose services, as I have said, only become valuable by a prolonged stay in the country. Setting aside all considerations of humanity, and even of justice to our gallant army, the question becomes one that may be answered by a reference to figures. Whether is it more economical to expend a few thousand pounds in rewards to experienced medical officers, or to sacrifice the lives of some hundreds of our brave soldiers? Your Lordship, I am satisfied, is not likely to allow any such

a calculation to be entered upon; and had you not considered the life of a fellow-creature of far more value than
any amount of money, you would never have ordered that
inquiry which has led to the valuable report now before
me.

Next in importance, if not even more important than
any considerations connected with the arrangements
of the Medical Staff, I would call your Lordship's
attention to the great, and I might almost say, criminal
negligence of the government, in not providing a sufficient
number of Chaplains for the Forces on Foreign Stations.
While a regiment continues in Great Britain or Ireland,
the men are made to attend divine service regularly at
some church or chapel on every Sunday throughout the
year; but the moment they are embarked on board ship
for Colonial service, all care for their souls' welfare is
entirely lost sight of.   There is not, in the whole of our
West India Possessions, a single church or chapel where
a regiment can be assembled to hear the Prayers of the
Church read, or the Gospel of Christ preached.   There is
not even a shed where they can meet to receive any
religious or moral instruction.   They are literally compelled to live without God in the world; and Sunday
becomes of all days the most distinguished for drunken-
ness and all manner of irregularity, and generally sends
more patients to the hospitals than all the other six days
of the week.   There is, it is true, with the early dawn of
every Sunday morning, what is generally, (I had almost
said, in mockery,) called a Church Parade.   The men
are assembled in front of their barracks, exposed to the
damp and noxious exhalations from the moist earth, and
the slanting beams of the rising sun; when some clergy-

man of the colony, in a hurried manner, reads over the prayers of the morning service, or perhaps only a part of them; and of what he does utter, few, if any of the soldiers can hear one word. The men are then dismissed, and the day is spent by the greater portion of them in listless idleness in their barrack-rooms, or in sleeping exposed to the currents of air in the verandas or corridors, while the more profligate crowd into the canteens and grog-shops to get drunk and quarrel with each other. From this Sabbath idleness, and these Sunday broils, arise many of the diseases which prove most fatal in the Colonies.

The troops stationed in any Colony are now scarcely sufficient for the ordinary routine of duties required. Even when the strength of the garrison is complete, the men are seldom more than two nights in bed; but when from sickness, or the punishment of culprits by solitary or other confinement, the duty becomes so severe, and especially upon the good men of a regiment, that they have scarcely one night in bed, they become exhausted, fall ill, and are cut off, while the guilty and profligate escape. How often have I heard men of good principles, and still struggling against the inroads of sin, and even many who had fallen away, complain of this cruel abandonment of all concern for their spiritual welfare. In sickness there was no one to afford them consolation; in distress they could find no comforter; they never could approach the House of God, and no one came to invite them to do well or to prevent them from doing evil. Solitary confinement, or hard labour, were rather a relief than a punishment. Indeed, their regular military duties were often more severe than any chastisement a court-martial could inflict, and hence crimes were often committed, that what was called punishment might ensue. Can we wonder at the iniquity that prevails, or at the sickness and mortality that follow a life of such reckless indifference to all the rules and moral obligations that usually regulate the conduct of men even in the lowest state of civilization, and are sufficient often to beget a total disregard of all military subordination, and even contempt of death itself?

My Lord, the awful crimes that are daily and hourly committed by our soldiers in the West Indies, and of which the people of Great Britain know nothing, will yet stand in fearful array against those who have withheld the means of lessening, if not altogether of preventing their occurrence. There was a time when our rulers considered it right and proper, that every regiment should have its own pastor, and even in the height of the Peninsular war every brigade had its chaplain ; but now, over the whole extent of the Windward and Leeward Island command there is only one military chaplain, and he is stationed in an Island (Trinidad) where his services are perhaps less required than in any other. Yet, even he has no place where he can perform Divine Service to the troops in that island, and during the many years that my friend, the Reverend David Evans, has been condemned to reside in that most unhealthy spot, I am not aware that he has ever been able to preach a sermon to the troops. It could only be done under the scorching rays of a Tropical Sun, and this no human constitution could withstand.

The late illustrious and amiable Duke of York procured for every regiment a supernumerary non-commis-

sioned officer, who was to act as schoolmaster to the
children of the soldiers; but, in the West Indies, as there
are no churches neither are there any school-houses. In
most instances, therefore, the children grow up in igno-
rance of all religious feelings or moral principles, but
abundantly instructed in all the profligacy and vices of
the barrack-room; there is scarcely any wickedness with
which they are not made acquainted from their most
tender years. Those who have gone in infancy to the
West Indies with their parents, too often return, after
a ten years' residence, as ignorant as the beasts that
perish; already full grown men in sin, and quite prepared
for any iniquity.

Now, my Lord, if it should be considered too expen-
sive for this *poor* country to return to the good old
system of giving every regiment its own chaplain, you
might surely manage to get squeezed into the Estimates,
a sum sufficient to provide a regular clergyman for our
principal Colonies in the West Indies. A clergyman,
who should have no other duty than to attend to the
spiritual wants of the garrison. To see that the children
were carefully instructed, and to assist in their instruction, and to visit the sick. In every Colony, my Lord,
there ought to be, and I venture to say, *must* be, a Military Church, where the soldiers can assemble and meet
together for religious purposes; and the provision of
them, I would add, may, with proper management, be
made at a very trifling expense, either to the mother
country or to the Colony. Wood can be had for the cut-
ting, and there is not a regiment in the service without
artificers sufficient to construct a building such as is
required. To do so, would not only afford amusement,

but procure health for the men. Experience has fully proved, that the more men are kept in employment (even within the Tropics) the healthier they become; and the best conditioned men in the garrison at St. Ann's, Barbados, are " *the hard labour gangs*," that is, the culprits who have been sentenced to hard labour. To many, if not to all, it is a boon rather than a punishment to be so employed ; they have just that degree of indolent exercise during the day, which secures for them a sound sleep during the night ; they are prevented from inflaming their blood with ardent spirits, and have abundance of food. The prison is often more comfortable than the guard-room, while there is no troublesome corporal to rouse them from their slumbers " to walk the sentry's weary round," during the silent watches of the night, exposed to all the torments and annoyances of the clouds of mosquitos that are then in search of blood.

Without the aid of religion, human laws and human punishments avail but little in restraining the evil passions of men ; and, if only as regards the safety of our own persons and property, a pious and benevolent pastor is of far more importance in a military community than any dreaded Provost-Martial. Many will act well from their love and respect for the one, who would disregard all consequences, and sink into crime, merely to show that they had no fear of the other. The infidel is always a coward, and the freethinker is never to be trusted. In all ages, and under all circumstances, religion has been made the foundation upon which all other rules and regulations have been based for the government of man— without it all human laws are vain. The heathen acted well from a dread of giving offence to his implacable deities, or that he might gain their favour for some selfish purpose ; and the rulers of such people took care to paint the wrath of the gods as terrible beyond what any mind could conceive, and their favour as worthy of any sacrifice. It remained, my Lord, for a people professing a belief in the precepts of the Gospel, by their openly acknowledging the truth of the Christian dispensation, to show by their practice and conduct, that they set at nought the wisdom of ages, and considered the experience of four thousand years as an idle dream. We are that people—we have been trying to keep in subjection our soldiers in the Colonies by the terror of human laws, and to prevent crime by the dread of temporal punishment. But have we succeeded? I could adduce a thousand instances to prove the contrary.

We are told in a book, which I am sure your Lordship reads, that " SIN BROUGHT DEATH INTO THE WORLD;" and I maintain that more than one-half of all the sickness and mortality that prevail among our troops in the West Indies originate from their crimes—crimes which can only be lessened or prevented by a greater attention to the moral and religious instruction of the men.

By procuring for them a due supply of the bread of life, which is as necessary for their souls' health and moral government, as were the fresh meat rations which your Lordship procured for their bodily comfort, you will more effectually diminish the great loss of life which is annually experienced in these Colonies than by any other measures you can possibly adopt.

There are many circumstances of minor importance that equally demand your attention, but these will come more properly under consideration in my analysis of the different sections of the Report itself, to which I now proceed.

In the first section there is nothing that calls particularly for any remark. The description of the Windward and Leeward command is accurately given, and the number and character of the several islands fairly stated; it is, however, to be regretted, that in the Health Returns, a greater attention has not been paid to the geological features of our several Colonies. In the West Indies, disease is not only greatly modified by the seasons of the year, and prevailing state of the weather, but is also affected by many peculiarities in regard to the locality of the barracks, the irregularities of the earth's surface, and more especially by the varieties of soil and state of cultivation in the several islands and around our our military stations.

The Medical Reports which I examined in the Inspector's office at Barbados,—and I went over a period of more than twenty years,—convinced me that fevers of one kind or another, were by far the most prevalent and most fatal diseases throughout the whole command. This agrees with Captain Tulloch's Report ; and, it is certainly somewhat remarkable, that though less frequent in the islands than on the main land of South America, they have proved far more malignant when they have occurred in any one of the islands, than they have ever yet been in British Guiana. It is also rather singular, that the average annual mortality throughout the command for a great number of years, has varied so very little in ordinary seasons. It has frequently happened that all the Colonies have been healthy except one, and yet the sickness and mortality in that one have been sufficient to bring the total number of deaths to the nearly common annual average. It seems also to be proved that in most of the islands, when much rain fell in summer and autumn, the winter and spring were generally healthy, though in some few districts, the contrary takes place. While Dr. Fergusson, of Windsor, was at the head of the Medical Department in the West Indies, he was at great pains to investigate every locality, and to satisfy himself of the circumstances by which disease was either engendered or affected. It would have added considerably to the value of this Report, had Captain Tulloch made more use of the doctor's scientific observations.

Our several Colonies, my Lord, differ so materially in physical aspect, local peculiarities, and geological formations, that, in all that regards the health of the human race, a separate chapter is required for each. Nay, so far does the influence of locality prevail, that the management of healthy troops, and the treatment of the sick, which are proper at one station, even in the same Colony, will sometimes be most improper at another. It requires, therefore, an investigation far more searching than can ever be made from any mass of general Reports or official Returns, and one that must be conducted, as Dr. Fergusson did his, on the spot, before your Lordship can obtain any sound data on which to found " efficient means for diminishing the great loss of life annually experienced in these Colonies."

The extent of barrack accommodation has been greatly enlarged since 1830, and the condition of many has been much improved ; still, there is not within the whole command a single station that might not be altered for the better, except, I believe, the new barracks built

under the direction of Sir Benjamin D'Urban, at Eve
Leary in British Guiana.

Captain Tulloch has given us a Table to show the
dimensions of barrack room, and a scale of accommodation with hammocks, prior to 1827, at Tobago, which, as
he states, was then one of the best in the command; that
extent did not exceed 22 or 23 inches in breadth to each
man! or, about 250 cubic feet of space. They have now
from 350 to 400 cubic feet, which he gives as the average
space to each soldier in the barracks of this command.

Though there is not much to complain of, as regards
space in any of the barracks, there are many of them
still most improperly built; and, as regards those of
Tobago, whatever space may be allowed for each man,
they will always prove unhealthy. Perched on the top
of a steep hill, and on the lee-side of an extensive swamp,
from which every exhalation of marsh poison is wafted by
the trade wind to Fort King George, we cannot wonder,
that the garrison here is always decimated, and often
nearly annihilated.

Captain Tulloch's second Table, my Lord, is intended
to show the number of white troops that were employed
in the command during each year, from 1817 to 1836
inclusive, with the admissions into hospital and number
of deaths in each year. In his third Table, page 11, we
have a similar statement for the black troops. I have
been at the trouble of making a comparison between the
strength as stated in these returns, and that given in
a return from the Adjutant-General's Office, dated the
25th of March, 1834, and the difference is so great, that
I think it calls for some notice.

Captain Tulloch states the number of white troops in

1823 to be 3264, and the black troops for the same year 2359, total 5623. Sir John M'Donald gives the whole strength, including Colonial corps, with officers, non-commissioned officers, and rank and file as 4565. In 1827 the white troops, according to Captain Tulloch, were 4310, the black 1543, total 5863; while Sir John M'Donald gives the total at 5411. In no one year of the twenty can I make the two returns agree.

From a Return which I made out at Barbados in 1834, I find that the total number of cases admitted into all our hospitals in the West Indies in five years, from 1823 to 1827 inclusive, was 47,005; and the total number of deaths during these years, 1783. That in four years, from 1829 to 1832 inclusive, 39,122 cases were admitted, and 1318 died. For the first period, Captain Tulloch gives the admission as 47,079, so that here we very nearly agree, and in the number of deaths we are the same, viz., 1467 white troops, and 316 black, total 1783. In the second period, the Captain gives only 38,826 as admitted, and the deaths in the white troops 1111, and in the black 236, making the total 1347, or 29 more than I have made them. Of the 1783 deaths in the first period, or in the five years from 1823 to 1827 inclusive, 697 were cases of fever; and in the second period, from 1829 to 1832 inclusive, 418 of the total number of 1318, are marked as deaths from fever in my return.

It appears further from Captain Tulloch's Tables, that every soldier was under medical treatment for one disease or another once in every six and a half months, and that from eighty to eighty-five of every thousand of the troops in the command have died annually during the last twenty years; or, that our actual loss by death has

been about one-eleventh of our military force during that
period. My average gives only one-fifteenth. The mortality among the troops in the West Indies, he states
to be six times greater than in the United Kingdom,
though the admissions into hospital are only double.
The total admissions in twenty years are stated to be
164,935, the deaths 6803. The cases from fever were
more than three eighths of the whole number, and the
deaths from fever amount to very nearly one half of our
total loss.

I am most desirous of calling your Lordship's serious
attention to these facts, because, if a remedy can be
found which will arrest the progress of so general and
so fatal a disease, it becomes, in my humble opinion, a
matter of national importance, to make it generally
known. And that such a remedy has been discovered, I
do most firmly and conscientiously believe—one, that is
of far more value than any preparation of the *quinquinas*,
or what is usually called the Spanish or Jesuits' bark, and
one whose powers have now been sufficiently proved to
warrant its being ordered by authority in the treatment
of fever throughout the whole range of our West India
and other Colonies.

It was my good fortune to serve for about twelve
months in the Colony of British Guiana, where, as Captain
Tulloch's returns show, fever is far more prevalent than
in any other British Colony ; and where, during what
was called the sickly season, from June till November,
our hospitals were crowded with every form of the disease.
I found that the *sulphate of quinine*, which in Europe and
in some of the other colonies had been most efficacious
in checking the fever, failed entirely in producing any

remission of the symptoms in most of our cases, and when pushed to any extent led to sufferings of an anomalous and distressing kind, that aggravated, rather than lessened, the violence of the febrile action. In almost every variety of the colonial epidemic, the irritability of the stomach is such as to preclude the exhibition of the bark in substance, or even in the form of a decoction or infusion. Under these circumstances, I was induced to have recourse to a remedy which had already become known in the Colony, and was much talked of as Dr. Warburg's Fever Drops.

I got introduced to the Doctor, who had been resident in Demerara for several years, as a civil practitioner; and soon discovered that he was a physician of very superior talents and a man of keen observation; a botanist of some distinction and well acquainted with modern chemistry; and, above all, that he was an enthusiast in science, and often spent months with the Indians in the woods in search of knowledge. The fever drops about which I was anxious, he assured me were prepared from plants, the virtues of which he had ascertained during his sojournings with the native tribes; and he laid before me evidence which proved that the reports I had heard were not exaggerations. I therefore did not hesitate to direct my able assistant, Dr. Gibson, to give the medicine a fair trial in the regimental hospital of the 25th regiment. It was administered in about fifty of our worst cases, and under my own eye, with the most perfect success. Dr. Warburg offered to supply us gratuitously with any quantity we might require, but I felt that as I was not allowed to purchase it for the use of the troops, I had no right to encroach upon the liberality of any individual for the benefit of the public, and was therefore compelled to decline his offer. I did not fail, however, to record what I had witnessed in my official Medical Reports, and I accepted of a supply, which was sent to the Director-General, with a request that trial might be made of its effects in the fevers of Gibraltar and the Mediterranean. I have not heard what the result has been, and possibly it may never have been tried.

There is generally and, I would say, very properly a great disinclination, on the part of the regular profession, to prescribe remedies of which we know not the composition; but when experience has fully established the character of any drug, or combination of drugs, and it is fairly ascertained that the exhibition of any remedy is uniformly followed by the same effects, in the treatment of the same class of diseases, we are perfectly warranted in adopting it in our *Materia Medica.* And if it shall be found to surpass all other remedies in the cure of that disease, we would, I conceive, become most criminal if we did not employ it, though the preparation may be kept secret. In this case, however, Dr. Warburg is too liberal and enlightened a physician to have any desire for secrecy. He has been at great trouble and great expense in bringing to perfection these invaluable drops, and in distributing them to all quarters of the globe, that they might be tried, and their success or failure in all cases of fever fairly and candidly reported. And, as it now appears, that whenever they have been tried they have succeeded, he thinks he is entitled to some remuneration for the time he has consumed, and the money he has expended, in procuring so important a benefit for the whole human race; and that too before he puts others

upon an equality with himself in regard to its preparation. I confess, my Lord, there is justice in this;
and when your Lordship again refers to the appalling
number of cases, 717 in every thousand, of the mean
strength of our whole troops! and of the mortality that
ensues, I trust you will not feel that I have dwelt too
long upon a matter, which promises to be of such vital
importance in the future treatment of our gallant soldiers,
who are subjected to the fearful ravages of West India
fever.

Taking all the classes of fever together, the medical
returns show, that only one out of every twenty admitted into hospital dies, but in some of the classes the
mortality is stated to be as high as one in nine; and in
the class called *Icteroedes* it is said to be one in every two
and a half. In the only instance in which I had an
opportunity of witnessing this aggravated form of the
bilious remittent, *one* only of the five patients seized
escaped.

Next to fever, diseases of the stomach and bowels
were the most frequent; but I believe your Lordship
has already found a remedy (*which is no secret*) for these
complaints. The additional fresh meat rations which,
through your means, were procured for the troops in this
command, have not only reduced the number of bowel
complaints, but have rendered their effects very much less
fatal. There is, however, one cause of such complaints
which I cannot pass over in silence; a cause from which
have originated many of the most severe and fatal cases
of dysentery, and some of the worst cases of diseases of
the lungs; and it is, my Lord, that *careless, uncomfortable,
and crowded manner in which regiments, or detachments of*

*regiments, have generally been conveyed from one colony to
another.* Men, women, and children, are all huddled
together upon the deck of the army vessel, or of some
less comfortable schooner: they often have not even
standing room, and are kept in this condition very frequently for one or two days and nights; as, unless it
be from Barbados to Grenada, or St. Vincents, the
voyage is seldom accomplished in less time*. They are
thus exposed to the chills and heavy dews of the night, or
to deluges of rain, alternately, with the burning and
scorching rays of the tropical sun during the day, in a
state of wretchedness and filth which it is not possible
to describe, and without being able to observe even the
common decencies of life. However healthy they may
have been when they embarked, it generally happens, if
the voyage has been at all lengthened, that many land
already labouring under acute dysentery, or inflammation
of the lungs; and that more are seized with these complaints immediately after their arrival, or with the colony
fever, to which the previous exhaustion has rendered
them peculiarly obnoxious.

There is an opinion, my Lord, which has been
entertained by many, and officially pronounced by some,
that removal from one colony to another was prejudicial
rather than of benefit to the health of the troops. Captain Tulloch professes himself unable to give an opinion
on this point. I had made up my mind that this could
not be the case; for though no fact is more firmly esta-

* While correcting this proof sheet, the account has just reached
me of the sufferings and loss of property of the head-quarters of the
14th Regiment from shipwreck, on their removal from Antigua; so that
the system is still continued.

blished, than that in some of the islands and stations for
the troops the average mortality is much greater than in
others, and, therefore, that the whole command may be
divided into what are called healthy and unhealthy stations; and that, however much casual circumstances, or
atmospheric changes, may for a time alter the character
of any one particular island, or military post, yet such
alteration is only temporary, while complaints of a specific
class will always prevail universally in the permanently
unhealthy islands. My opinion had been formed long
before I ever saw the West Indies, or had any intention
of visiting these colonies; yet I felt not the less anxious
that it should be confirmed, or otherwise refuted, by data
that should be free from all bias, and that must carry with
them a perfect degree of conviction, one way or the other.

I investigated the Returns for a great number of
years,—followed the movements, and noted the casualties of several regiments, during the whole of their stay
in the windward and leeward command,—and it appeared
even to me rather surprising, how uniformly all the
returns I examined supported each other, and how satis-
factorily they proved these great leading facts, namely,
*that the more frequently a regiment has been moved from one
island to another, or from one station to another*, in the
same island or colony, during its residence within the
command, *the fewer men it has lost; and that the most
stationary corps have always lost the greatest number of
men.* I shall only intrude upon your Lordship with the
history of two or three regiments.

Commencing with 1824, I took the 27th, 35th, and
93rd regiments. I found that during this year the 27th
regiment had arrived in the command, after a three years'

seasoning in the garrison of Gibraltar; the 35th had already been three years within the tropics; and the 93rd had just arrived from Ireland. The 35th and 93rd were quartered for the next two years in Barbados,—a healthy station;—the 27th at Demerara,—an unhealthy one. The 35th lost only thirty-seven men, while the 93rd lost sixty, and the 27th a hundred and seventeen. Here, I certainly thought, there was a strong proof of the advantage of the men having become accustomed to the climate, as, in the same garrison, the casualties of the newly arrived regiment were nearly double the number of those in the corps, that had had three years' seasoning. In 1826, the 35th regiment was moved to St. Lucia and Dominica; the 93rd to Antigua and St. Kitt's, while the 27th was allowed to remain in British Guiana. This year the 35th lost thirty-four men, and the 93rd only eighteen; the 27th not less than fifty. In 1827, it was found necessary to remove the 27th regiment to St. Vincents and Grenada, but the other two remained stationary. The deaths in the 27th are this year reduced from fifty to thirty-three, while in the 35th, the second year of its residence in St. Lucia and Dominica, they are increased from thirty-four to seventy-five, while the 93rd lost not more than in the former year, viz., eighteen. In 1828, there was no change of any of these corps, and I find the mortality stands thus:—the 27th, in a healthy station, lost thirty-five men; the 35th regiment, in a most unhealthy one, only twenty-one; and the 93rd lost nineteen in two of the most healthy islands in the command. In 1829, they also continued stationary. The deaths in the 27th regiment were this year twenty-five; in the 35th regiment forty-five; and in the 93rd they amounted to twenty-eight; proving, as I maintain, that their being so long stationary was beginning to take effect. In 1830, however, the whole were changed. The 27th and 35th regiments went to Barbados; the 93rd to St. Lucia and Dominica: the 27th lost only fourteen men; the 35th lost thirty-five; but the 93rd had to bury fifty-nine, the effect of climate, and certainly not of the movement. During these seven years the 27th regiment lost two hundred and seventy-four men, notwithstanding the preparation they had undergone by a previous three years' residence at Gibraltar; while the 93rd, direct from Ireland, lost only two hundred and two in the same period. And the 35th, which, with these seven years, had completed their ten years' service in the command, lost two hundred and fifty-seven.

I next took the 25th and 86th regiments; they both arrived in the command in 1826. The 25th, during the seven years that it remained stationary in British Guiana, lost two hundred and eighty-nine men; while the 86th, which, during these years had two or three moves, first from Barbados to Antigua and St. Kitt's, and, in 1828, (when they both had two years' seasoning,) from thence to British Guiana, lost only two hundred and sixteen men. The 1st battalion of the Royals affords another striking proof of what I have advanced. This steady and well-disciplined corps arrived at Barbados in 1826, and remained in that island for nearly two years, losing only seventeen men; (Captain Tulloch's Table says twenty-seven.) In 1828, it was moved to Trinidad and Tobago, where it remained stationary for four years, losing not less than a hundred and sixty-three men; (Captain Tulloch, a hundred and seventy.) The number of deaths in the fourth year of their residence was nearly the double of what occurred during their second year. From Trinidad, in 1832, they were moved to St. Lucia and Dominica, stations reckoned the most unhealthy of any in the command; but even with this drawback the movement proved so advantageous that they lost only thirty-three (Captain Tulloch thirty-eight) during that year, when, in the previous year at Trinidad, they had lost forty. And, I again repeat, that the mortality which has been so frequently attributed to the movement was, in most instances, solely owing to the very irregular and improper manner in which their movements were carried into effect.

It cannot, therefore, my Lord, be too strongly impressed upon the minds of the general officers, intrusted with the command of our troops in the West Indies, the great importance of adopting some fixed rule, with regard to the changing of the regiments from one station to another. No regiment should ever be allowed to remain longer in any one island or colony than two years; and our ships of war upon the station afford every facility for such removals, without any expense to the country, and without any of those distressing scenes of misery, and shipwreck, and exposure to the inclemency of the weather, which have hitherto led to so much sickness and mortality. If some fixed regulation was once adopted and strictly adhered to, both officers and men would know the extent of their misery in a bad cantonment, and the limit of their pleasures in a good one. The moral effect of such a certainty would have a powerful influence upon the health of both; their sufferings would be endured with patience and resignation, while their spirits would be sustained with hope, and even their pleasures would be enjoyed with a contentment and moderation that would greatly check their running into excess.

We know from the best of all sources, my Lord, that "hope deferred maketh the heart sick," and it is to the uncertainty and inconsistency, which apparently have too frequently prevailed in the changes and removals of the troops in this command, that I chiefly attribute those occasional explosions of disease which, in many instances, have proved so fatal. Whenever the exigencies of the service will admit of it, the comforts, the conveniences, and even the harmless pleasures of the soldier, should ever form the chief concern of the good and humane commanding officer: and whoever has witnessed the baneful effects of that callous indifference with which, I regret to say, the feelings of the men serving in the West Indies are sometimes treated, and the careless apathy with which their health and their lives are too often regarded, will feel no astonishment at the great loss of life annually experienced in these colonies. In Jamaica the troops ought to change their quarters once in every year.

I have now, my Lord, brought before you some of the most important causes of disease in our West India Colonies, and have pointed out the remedies which ought to be applied, and which are perfectly within your reach. If the measures I have suggested are adopted and carefully followed up, it will soon be found that sickness has decreased, and that the annual mortality has greatly diminished. But while our barracks continue placed on the tops of mountains, and the towns which the soldier has to frequent are situated at the base of these mountains, we must lay our account for a plentiful supply of chest complaints. Most of the diseases of the lungs, under whatever category they may be placed in Captain Tulloch's tables, arise from inflammatory action induced by the soldiers having to mount a steep ascent to get at their barracks, and where, on their arrival, overcome with heat and exhaustion, they expose their half-covered bodies to the chilling draughts of air that sweep through the galleries where they throw themselves down and fall asleep. As this is not a medical treatise, I shall not stop to annoy your Lordship with a reference to those diseases which are of rarer occurrence, and certainly of minor importance. Their number is, no doubt, considerable, yet they are seldom dangerous; for while the deaths from fevers, and from diseases of the stomach and bowels, and of the liver and lungs, amount to 6058 in the course of twenty years, our loss from all other diseases during the same length of time does not exceed 745 individuals.

I have already called your Lordship's attention to the difference which exists between the War Office Returns, as given by Captain Tulloch, and those from the Horse Guards, as given by General Macdonald. In no one year do these returns agree as to the strength of our troops in the command, and in twenty years, the Captain has 25,000 more than are certified for by the Adjutant General. This is a matter that requires explanation; for if in returns from two public offices, both supposed to be correct, we find a wide difference, what faith can we put in the calculations made from such uncertain data? The Captain, from merely enumerating the tables of figures as they stand in the Medical Returns, has produced results that certainly do not accord with the opinions pre-

viously entertained on some points of medical jurispru-
dence; but when we come to consider the thousand
contingencies that affect the quotation of numbers merely,
we shall find little reason to put any faith in an arithme-
tical problem.

In his description of British Guiana, Captain Tulloch
is tolerably correct, but he has copied apparently from
some old Medical Report, as *Porter's Hope* has not been
a military station for the last eight or nine years. He
ought to have set forth more fully the excellence of the
new barracks and hospitals, built under the superintendence of Sir Benjamin D'Urban; they are by far the
best in the whole command. The hospitals, when they
were building, were, I believe, within 150 yards of the
sea, but they are now two or three miles distant from it.

For many years after this Dutch province came into
our possession, it was not only considered, but certainly
was, the most unhealthy of all our Colonies. Few men
ever survived a three years' residence on its muddy shores,
and Demerara was emphatically termed "*the wet grave of
Europeans.*" Yet when I came to examine the subject on
the spot, and to look into the details and reports that had
been left by my predecessors, who had had charge of the
health of the troops from the commencement of our
occupancy, I found that the great mortality which had
occurred was not so much owing to the climate, or state
of the Colony, as to the wretched barracks, or close shut
up prisons, in which our troops were lodged. These dun-
geons were not only deficient as to space, but during the
night were so closely shut up, that the men could scarcely
breathe. The open holes, called windows, were then covered with wooden shutters, that excluded both wind and

rain, and were emphatically designated by the men *as the suffocaters*. If we take the mortality as given for the last eight years, during which the new barracks have been occupied, and the remainder of the old ones improved, and compare it with the preceding eight years, when great improvements and better arrangements had even then been made at all the old stations, we shall be able to form some estimate of the importance of proper barrack accommodation to the health of our troops. In eight years, from 1821 to 1828 inclusive, the total strength of our white troops in the Colony was 6639, and of these 764 died. From 1829 to 1836 inclusive, when the *suffocaters* had been abolished, and the D'Urban system adopted, I find the total strength to have been 8016 white troops, and the deaths in that period are only 489! The mortality at Berbice has always been greater than at Demerara, since the new barracks were occupied; yet as Berbice had for many years superior accommodation for the troops than existed at George Town, the average which Captain Tulloch has taken for twelve years, would lead us to believe that our military stations in Berbice were more healthy than in Demerara. But mere figures, I again repeat, cannot be relied on when health and disease are under consideration.

I am not satisfied, my Lord, of the correctness of the data upon which Captain Tulloch has made some of his calculations as regards this Colony. One or two of his returns, I know of a certainty, are not accurate. In his table, page 15, he tells us that the number of white troops in British Guiana in 1834 was 1228, and that of these sixty-five died. That the black troops amounted to 189, and that *five* died during the year.

Now, my Lord, I have before me my own Annual

Report, as principal medical officer of the Colony for that year, with the returns that accompanied it; and the annexed table will sufficiently prove how much the Captain has been misled.

DETAILED TABLE, showing the MORTALITY in the several CLASSES of PERSONS belonging to the MILITARY ESTABLISHMENT in BRITISH GUIANA, for the Year 1834.

CLASSES OF PERSONS.	Average Number of each Class.	Average Number of Deaths.	Proportion of Deaths.	REMARKS.
British officers	46	1	1 in 46	General staff officers, Royal Artillery, 25th and 86th Regiments.
Officers' wives	21	..	..	
Officers' children	28	..	..	
British serjeants	59	7	1 in $8\frac{3}{7}$	
British corporals	52	3	1 in $17\frac{1}{3}$	
British soldiers	948	40	1 in $23\frac{28}{40}$	
Soldiers' wives	59	6	1 in $9\frac{5}{6}$	
Soldiers' children	137	5	1 in $27\frac{2}{5}$	
African soldiers	62	..	..	1st West India Regiment.
African women	23	..	..	1st West India Regiment, and military labourers.
Negro children	43	..	..	
African labourers	89	3	1 in $29\frac{2}{3}$	Military labourers.
General Average	1,567	65	1 in $24\frac{7}{65}$	

Demerara, 21st January, 1835.

From this table, your Lordship will perceive, that, including officers, and men, women, and children, of all colours, and of all denominations, the total number of persons was 1567, and of these only sixty-five died; and as I do not suppose Captain Tulloch intended to include women and children upon the strength of either the white or the black troops, he is in error both as to strength and mortality. The number of the white troops, including officers and men, was never more than 1105, and the black soldiers and labourers 151. The deaths in the first were fifty-one, and in the latter three, total fifty-four instead of seventy, as stated in the Report. If in one year we find so great a discrepancy between the actual facts and the *Reported* statements, I fear, my Lord, we must take the calculations of the gallant Captain in some instances, as only approximating to the truth.

The next Colony that engages the attention of our able statist is Trinidad. The Island is well described, and its military stations accurately pointed out. But I question, if there are other five acres of habitable land in the whole Island so very unsuitable for a military station, as regards the health of the troops, as that which has been chosen in the parish of St. James. It is on the verge of a very extensive plain, and nearly at the base of a steep mountain. Instead of standing on "a gently sloping plain," the barracks are placed in what may be called a hollow basin, surrounded on all sides, but one, by higher land, and are so little elevated above the waters of the Gulf of Paria, that, notwithstanding the sandy nature of the soil it is at all times saturated with moisture. There can be no perfect drainage; and the immediate vicinity of the Cocorite swamp, together with "their exposure to the sudden gusts of wind which sweep through the deep ravines, or gullies, loaded with moisture, and the noxious exhalations from a large tract of uncultivated ground in their rear," will ever render them a most unhealthy and improper residence for European troops. Instead of being elevated upon pillars, as in British Guiana, the basement story has been closely built up, and converted into store-rooms, or cellars, and so powerfully does the miasma accumulate in these dungeon-like apartments, that at times every soldier in the lower story becomes affected with the fever. There is also a mountain stream which descends through one of the deep ravines, and half encircles the barrack square. For several months of every year the channel of this stream appears perfectly dry, and during these months the marsh poison is distilled in such abundance, that the banks of this river along its whole course become unfit for the residence of man.

The hospital is certainly placed upon the most elevated portion of the barrack square, but nevertheless is low compared with the hills behind it, and is almost embosomed in the impenetrable bush, while the densely wooded mountains hang over it on every side but one. Orange Grove, the more ancient barrack station upon this plain, is nearer to the Capital (Port of Spain); but here, too, a low damp situation, on the margin of another pestilential mountain stream, has been chosen, and the buildings have been pushed as close under the lee of the mountains, and into the bush, as it is possible; so that there is no free circulation of air to dissipate the exhalations when they do accumulate, or to dilute the poison, which at certain seasons is generated in such abundance as to render the locality so extremely unhealthy that it cannot be tenanted by white troops. Luckily, the buildings at Orange Grove are now in such a state of dilapidation that they can scarcely be tenanted by any troops; and I hope, my Lord, that common sense will at last be allowed to dictate, and that a new locality will be chosen, (and there are a thousand eligible situations in this extensive plain,) and suitable barrack accommodation be provided, after the style of the Eve Leary barracks, in British Guiana. If this is done, I venture to assure your Lordship, that Trinidad will become as healthy a station for British troops as any in the Caribbean Archipelago.

St. Joseph's, situated about seven miles from Port of Spain, in the interior of the Island, will always be unhealthy from being situated on a high table-land, surrounded on three sides by the great Eastern marsh, and backed by lofty mountains, that attract the poison from that marsh, and which at times is stopped in its progress, or finds a halting place upon that table-land, and there commits its frightful ravages.

Last summer the mortality at St. Joseph's was truly alarming. Fortunately, however, the buildings here are so old and rotten, that new barracks must be provided somewhere. I am quite satisfied, that if brought lower down, and removed to a distance from the mountain torrent, kept just so much above the level of the plain as to admit of perfect drainage, and a canal cut between them and the marsh, they too will be found tolerably healthy.

Of late years, and since the arrangement was made for furnishing the garrison of Tobago from the regiment stationed in Trinidad, a considerable portion of the mortality at the latter station has arisen from disease contracted in the former Island. At Tobago, as Captain Tulloch has shown, the mortality has been nearly double the rate which prevails throughout the whole of the windward and leeward command; and I am afraid, my Lord, it will ever continue to be so until Fort King George ceases to be a military station. While I was resident in Trinidad, several of the casualties which took place in the hospital of the 19th regiment, at St. James's, were men who had returned sick from the detachment at Tobago. The *Bacolette* swamp, which is within the distance of less than half a mile of the Fort, and as I have said, directly to windward, and which every year has been increasing in extent and in the virulence of its exhalations, is quite sufficient to account for that increase of sickness and mortality in this Island of late years, which the Captain in his Report attributes to some unknown cause. My own opinion is, that it is the locality of Fort King George, and not the climate of Tobago, that has become in any degree deteriorated; though the deposition of mud, and the formation of new land in the direction of Trinidad, and under the lee of the Basaltic Rocks that constitute the mountainous portion of this volcanic Island, may, and no doubt has, increased the quantity of noxious vapours that spread over the whole Island, and also increased their virulence. I do not learn, however, that any epidemic has since proved so fatal to the white inhabitants of the Colony, as that which prevailed in 1801; for though the yellow fever of 1820 was more destructive to our troops, it was not so generally to the Colonists, and therefore, as already stated, the apparent change for the worse in the climate of Tobago may be rather local than general.

The fevers of this Island have generally assumed a most malignant type, and happy will it be, my Lord, if by the introduction into general use of the remedy I have ventured to bring to your notice, we can stop the ravages of so fatal a malady. Between the middle of February and the 8th of July, 1820, as appears from a table given by Captain Tulloch, page 21, the detachment of the 4th regiment, consisting of six officers, 123 non-commissioned

officers and privates, eleven women, and six children,—a
total of 146 persons,—had 138 attacked with fever, and
of these 100 died.

The ratio of deaths annually among the white troops
in British Guiana for a period of twenty years is only
59·2 in the thousand of the mean strength. In Trinidad
it is 61·6, but in Tobago it is as high as 153, or, as
already said, double the rate which prevails throughout
the whole of the military stations in this command.

Grenada and St. Vincent's are both esteemed healthy
Colonies, though occasionally fever has raged with great
malignity. The mortality at Grenada has always been
greater than at St. Vincent's, in the proportion of 61 to
55 per thousand. In 387 deaths which occurred at
Grenada in twenty years, 165 were from fever; while at
St. Vincent's in the same period, though there were 408
deaths, 85 only were occasioned by fever. Having had
no opportunity of visiting either of these islands, I am
unable to offer any positive opinion as to the probable
cause of so remarkable a circumstance as the mortality
from fever in these two neighbouring islands being so
different. I imagine, however, that it possibly may
arise from the moisture in Grenada being kept near the
surface of the earth, and more powerfully acted upon by
the solar heat, and that in the centre of the island there
are several hill lakes. Grenada is a mass of solid rock,
over which, even in its most fertile valleys, a thin
stratum of earth has only as yet been spread; while the
ashes and porous tuffa or lava of the still active volcano of
St. Vincent's, have covered its more solid materials to a
considerable depth. In the one case, the water is rapidly
called back into the atmosphere, bringing with it the

poisonous miasmata that induce and render virulent
endemic fever; but in the other, it soon gets beyond the
influence of the sun, accumulates, and is conveyed to the
ocean in open or concealed channels. The whole Island,
(St. Vincent's,) we are told, is well watered by numerous
rivulets, but there is no mention of any lakes.

Of Barbados, I can speak with more certainty, having
well examined it in all its bearings. This island, as is well
known, is a mass of solid granite, cased with coral rock,
and which evidently has been raised from the bosom of
the deep, not by one effort of nature, but by a succession of
efforts. The Polypes that formed the pinnacle of Mount
Hillaby while it was yet under the wave, may have lived
some thousand years before the generations that built the
next terrace ; and conjecture is lost in imagining the
ages that may have elapsed since even the last raised
portions of this island assumed their present level. The
comminuted portions of the calcareous earth are in
general too scanty to admit of a luxuriant vegetation;
hence, most of the hills are naked and barren; but opposed
to what may be called the current of the ocean, or the
force of the waves, as impelled by the constant action of
the trade winds, the solid nucleus of Barbados, with its
adventitious covering, have assumed the form of a cres-
cent, with the points stretching to the north east and
south east, and forming a deep bay. In this bay the
muddy waters, checked in their course, were allowed to
deposit the earthy particles they had collected in their
progress ; and from these particles a considerable extent of
solid land has now been formed, of a nature entirely dis-
tinct from the great mass of the island—a pure alluvial
clay soil, mixed with the thousand and one substances

that are usually found in all such recent formations. The surface of this soil is covered with every variety of vegetation and forest trees. It has of course been broken up by the action of the rains, and is now formed into mimic mountains and sequestered valleys, abounding in mineral springs and asphaltic exudations; and, at one spot, affording the singular phenomena of a burning well.

If more attention was paid to the spiritual welfare of the troops, and greater care shown for their temporal comforts, St. Ann's would be as healthy a station as any in Europe. True, it is, there are times and seasons when sickness prevails to a great extent even here, but these are now of rare occurrence. There ought, and eventually *must* be, two regular chaplains commissioned for this garrison, a Protestant and a Roman Catholic; yes, my Lord, a Roman Catholic, for there are seldom fewer than three or four hundred soldiers professing that religion quartered here, and for many years there has not been a clergyman of that persuasion resident on the island.

On a late occasion, when a poor unfortunate wretch was condemned to be shot for a breach of military discipline, it was left to the humanity of a merchant of the colony, to freight a schooner at his own expense to bring a priest from a neighbouring island to attend the criminal in his last moments. Are we a Christian people, and can allow such things to pass unheeded? The Protestant clergyman, who is allowed a pittance from the army extraordinaries, (seven shillings and sixpence *per diem*,) as garrison chaplain, has no means of discharging the sacred duties of his office. He does read the Morning Prayers to the men in front of their barracks on a Sunday morning, and may occasionally marry a couple, or christen a child; but as to preaching a sermon, or holding any religious communion with the idle and reckless soldiery, these are entirely out of the question.

Now, my Lord, in this very garrison there is a building that has cost the country a great deal of money, which at present is lost to all useful purposes, but which, at an expense of another hundred pounds, might be converted into a most comfortable and commodious church, capable of holding fifteen hundred men, and where the Morning and Evening service might be regularly and devoutly performed. This building, my Lord, is known as the Ordnance-Hospital. There are never more than *five* or *six* patients at any one time in this hospital, and for these there is more than an abundance of room in the general military hospital, and where, too, they can be attended with equal facility, and more advantage by their own medical officers.

What right, I would ask, can this branch of the service have to such useless magnificence? Why this special indulgence, which is without one advantage to the sick, when so large and well ordered a building might be converted to so important and useful a purpose as a church for the white troops on Sunday, and a school for their children during the other days of the week? The Protestant and the Roman Catholic might meet here at different hours, and in comfort and peace hear the glad tidings of salvation from the lips of their respective pastors, and this would have more effect upon their moral conduct, and tend more to preserve their health than all that has yet been done by military regulations or any dread of punishment. I implore your Lordship to give this matter a serious thought : you are not one to despise such counsel.

With regard to temporal comforts, I must again recur to the soldier's bedding. Their palliasses were stuffed with *the crude husks of the Indian corn,* a most filthy and unwholesome material. When five years ago, I made some stir about this matter, I was at last informed by the then Secretary of the Ordnance, that " Hair matresses had been ordered for the white troops in the West Indies." But have they been provided? Are the corn husks no longer in use at Barbados? and, have the plantain leaves been laid aside at Demerara? I hope I shall be informed that they are, but I have my doubts.

From Captain Tulloch's tables, it appears that bowel complaints are not only frequent, but most fatal among the troops situated in Barbados. How can it be otherwise, when men, women, and children are compelled to have recourse to the same open and filthy privies, where vermin are generated in millions, and often productive of most distressing and dangerous bowel complaints? Independent of the profligacy to which this leads, it shows such a total disregard for the common decencies of humanity, and tends so effectually to do away with all feeling of self-respect, that there is scarcely any inducement left for either class to act well. Besides, my Lord, at Barbados these *necessaries* are placed at such a distance from the barracks, that when they have to be visited during the night, or when the weather is unsettled, the individual who has risen from his bed in a state of profuse perspiration, is often so drenched with rain, that he returns shivering to his uneasy couch, and is either carried off in a day or two by acute dysentery, or is seized with inflammation of the liver or lungs, which, if they do not kill, soon render him totally unfit for the service, and he is invalided and sent home to die of lingering consumption or chronic hepatitis. Of 1401, the total deaths in twenty years at Barbados, 911 were from diseases of the lungs, the liver, and of the stomach and bowels, and only 282 from fever. If the commanding engineer were so disposed, a remedy could soon be found for the evil I am here complaining of, and one far more beneficial to the health of the troops, and more conducive to good moral conduct, than all the stone walls and iron barricades that can ever be built to keep them from the grog-shops.

Having no personal experience of St. Lucia, or of any of the other colonies, I am unable to offer any suggestions with regard to them.

The Tables, section 3, of Captain Tulloch's Report, distinctly show, that out of every thousand white troops there are eighty-seven constantly ineffective from sickness in the windward and leeward command, and only sixty-three in Jamaica, though the latter is by far the most unhealthy. But, as is well observed, three-fourths of the mortality in Jamaica being caused by fevers, which rapidly terminate, either in death or recovery, there is often a very great mortality, without the hospitals being in any degree more crowded than usual.

Before I conclude, my Lord, I would wish to call Captain Tulloch's attention to the apparent difference which exists between the number of deaths, as given by him in his Table 75, page 90, and that which I have given in the regiments whose movements I have stated in the foregoing pages. My numbers for the three first, are

taken from the Returns and Reports in the Inspector-
General's office at Barbados, where, if correctness is at
all to be expected, it ought to be found, for they are the
actual returns of the medical officer in charge of each
regiment, and are witnessed by the commanding officer.
The following Tables, in which I have put my numbers,
and those given by Captain Tulloch, in juxta position,
will show that there must be a considerable error somewhere.

Regiments.	Number of Deaths in each Year for 7 Years, from Barbados Returns.							Total in Seven Years.
	1824	1825	1826	1827	1828	1829	1830	
27th Regt.	70	47	50	33	35	25	14	274
35th Ditto.	20	17	34	75	21	45	35	247
93rd Ditto.	35	25	18	18	19	28	59	202

Regiments.	Number of Deaths in each Year from War Office Returns.							Total in Seven Years.
	1824	1825	1826	1827	1828	1829	1830	
27th Regt.	78	47	52	37	32	19	20	285
35th Ditto.	27	28	39	77	27	59	43	300
93rd Ditto.	16	18	19	20	21	32	57	183

The numbers, you will observe, seldom agree in any
year, and the totals, especially in the 35th regiment, are
very different in the two Returns. I am inclined to
believe that mine were fairly copied from the originals.
With regard to the 25th and 86th regiments, the numbers were taken from the Regimental Hospital Books,
and stand thus:—

Regiments.	Number of Deaths in each Year for 7 Years, from Regimental Returns.							Total in Seven Years.
	1828	1829	1830	1831	1832	1833	1834	
25th Regt.	35	92	29	42	42	27	22	289
86th Ditto.	46	28	29	19	23	25	46	216

Regiments.	Number of Deaths in each Year for 7 Years, from War Office Returns.							Total in Seven Years.
	1828	1829	1830	1831	1832	1833	1834	
25th Regt.	109	31	32	56	29	19	20	296
86th Ditto.	29	26	23	26	41	37	33	215

The total numbers come nearer to each other in this table than they do in the other, but still in no one year do they actually agree. As regards the first battalion of the Royals, our returns are more at variance.

Return of casualties in the 1st battalion of the Royal regiment for seven years:—

Regiment.	Number of Deaths in each Year for 7 Years, from Sir A. Halliday's Returns.							Total in Seven Years.
	1826	1827	1828	1829	1830	1831	1832	
1st Batt.	8	9	58	25	40	40	33	213

Regiment.	Number of Deaths in each Year for 7 Years, from Captain Tulloch's Returns.							Total in Seven Years.
	1826	1827	1828	1829	1830	1831	1832	
1st Batt.	9	18	60	27	42	41	38	235

As my numbers are taken from the Medical Returns, and as the Captain's are corrected from those in the War

Office, there will of course be some difference, yet not such, I imagine, as can account for what appears in the above Tables; one or other of us therefore must be in error.

I quite agree, my Lord, with what Captain Tulloch has stated as to the effects of acclimatization, and had satisfied myself long before I saw the results of his inquiry, that it was the *locality*, and not the *climate generally*, that principally affected the health of the troops. Still a great deal of the sickness, and not a little of the mortality that has occurred in regiments newly arrived in the West Indies, has arisen from the reckless indifference with which they have been too often sent to the very worst stations in the command, and kept there until, perhaps, the half or two-thirds of the whole corps had been lost.

I consider it of the very greatest importance to order that a regiment on its arrival within the tropics, should be kept for the first year at a healthy station, for there are many circumstances connected with a change, so sudden and so great, as regards the habits and feelings of the individuals, that are not only calculated to induce disease themselves during the first months of their residence, but still more to aggravate every symptom of any epidemic to which they may be exposed. So little attention do the higher authorities seem to have paid to what I would call the best interests of the British soldiers, and involving (as I believe these interests do) the welfare of the British Empire, that, without apparently any other reason than their own caprice, regiments have not only been sent out from England so as to arrive within the tropics at the most unhealthy period of the whole year, but immediately on their arrival, have been sent to those stations where sickness prevailed most at all seasons, and was probably then most malignant, and have been kept there, as I have just said, till more than the half had perished, and scarcely a man remained fit for duty.

In war time, my Lord, regiments must go when and where they are required, and their stations must be dependant upon the exigences of the service ; but since the peace, and during the period embraced in Captain Tulloch's Report, I am quite satisfied that had common sense and a trifling degree of reflection regulated our military arrangements as connected with the troops sent to, and kept serving in the West Indies, the mortality would have been lessened by at least one-third. And although I admit that men do not live longer, nor escape disease by any acclimatization in the West Indies, yet many, very many lives are lost that would have been saved, had the regiments not been sent immediately on their arrival into those localities where fever was already committing its ravages, and where it was impossible the men could escape the effects of the concentrated poison. The newly-arrived may not be so likely to catch the fever as is his debilitated and acclimated comrade, but when both become affected, it generally proves of a far more malignant type in the one than in the other, and the old resident will escape when the healthy and vigorous new comer is cut off.

It is, therefore, of the utmost consequence to keep men during what is very properly called their " seasoning fever," from the poisonous influences of any prevailing epidemic, for if this is not done, we shall find the mortality, in both officers and men, far beyond the average

of any other year of their residence, even at the most
unhealthy stations. That troops are likely to gain but
little immunity, from disease or mortality, by a prolonged
residence in the West Indies, is evident from the results
of the Captain's inquiry. Yet, I again assert that it
depends far more upon the station, whether disease and
death are more prevalent at the commencement of their
service or during its middle term, or near its close, than
upon any other circumstance

The Royals lost considerably more men in the third
and fourth years of their residence, because they were
quartered at Trinidad and Tobago, than they did in the
eighth and ninth, though they were thirteen months
of these years in St. Lucia, and only eleven at Barbados. The 25th lost three times the number of men during
the third year of their residence in the West Indies
that they did in the two first, and twice as many as they
did during the three last years of their stay. The 35th
lost as many men during four years that they were kept
in St. Lucia, (from the seventh to the tenth years of their
residence,) as they did in seven years that they were at
other stations in the windward and leeward command.
The 19th Foot, from being sent to Demerara, lost more
men in the first year of its residence in that Colony, and
in this command, than it did in the next four years,
though three times moved, and considerably more than
it did in the four last years of its stay, although
it garrisoned Trinidad and Tobago during these years.
The 86th lost nearly double the number of men in the
first nine months after their arrival at Berbice, (which
took place in the seventh year of their service in the
command,) than they did in any other of the ten years

they remained. The 93rd lost more men in twenty-two months at St. Lucia, (the eighth and ninth years of its service in the command,) than it did in nearly nine years that it was at other stations; and the mortality in the last year of its stay was not greater than during its first, which were both spent at Barbados. It, therefore, I repeat, depends far more upon the station occupied, than upon any other circumstances whatever, whether sickness and mortality prevail most at the commencement or at the end, or in any intermediate year of a regiment's stay in the West Indies.

One thing, however, is certain : if a regiment is sent to an unhealthy or sickly station, immediately on its arrival from Europe, the casualties will certainly be more numerous than if it had been sent to that station, after a year or two's seasoning at some healthy station. In proof of this I would mention, that the 19th during the first year after its arrival from England lost 108 at Demerara; the 27th from Gibraltar lost in its first year seventy-eight at the same station; and the 65th from Ireland lost fifty-five at Berbice; while the 67th, after seasoning for three years at Barbados and St. Kitt's, lost only thirty-three men during its first year in British Guiana; and the 69th, who had spent two months in Barbados, and three years in St. Vincent's, lost only thirty-five men in the first year, and seventeen in the second of their residence at Demerara.

There are, however, years of sickness in healthy as well as in unhealthy Colonies, when no previous seasoning can withstand the virulence of the epidemic : but, as a general rule, a regiment should never be sent to British

E

Guiana, St. Lucia, or to Dominica, until it has been one
or two years in the West Indies.

These remarks, my Lord, apply to Captain Tulloch's
first and second conclusions, and the result of my
experience stands thus:—Sickness and mortality, as I
repeat for the third time, depend more upon station than
period of service, and *cæteris paribus* fever is more malignant in the newly imported, and the mortality is greater,
than in those who have been some years in the command.
This, too, is the Captain's conclusion as regards Jamaica:
and his reasoning to my mind is perfectly satisfactory.
Captain Tulloch's remarks on the effects of diet, and the
result of his inquiries, prove the necessity of the measure
your Lordship adopted two years ago. On his examination of the diseases by which soldiers suffer to a greater
extent than the officers, I would only observe, that, with
regard to diseases of the lungs, notwithstanding improper
diet and impure air are, without doubt, most important
predisposing causes, and that to those the soldier is much
more exposed than the officer, yet the great and principal
exciting cause of most of the acute, and many of the
chronic, affections of the lungs, arise from what I have
already stated, namely,—the position of the barracks on
some lofty eminence. The officer is neither called upon
to make such frequent journeys up and down the mountain steep, nor to perform those that he does make in so
hurried and irregular a manner, as the soldier too often
has to do from over-staying his leave; and when his
blood is already heated, and the circulation increased by
his visits to the grog-shops, in which he has lingered to
the last moment. Besides, most officers are able to keep

a horse of one description or another, and are saved the fatigue and exertions of these steep ascents. In proof, I refer your Lordship to the Captain's Tables of these Diseases.

In British Guiana, where there is no such exciting cause as that referred to, the deaths from diseases of the lungs are only 112 or 6·4 per thousand of the mean strength of the troops in the Colony. In Trinidad it rises to 11·5; and at Tobago it is 11: but almost all the casualties, from diseases of the lungs in Trinidad, have been in men who returned convalescent, or unfit for duty, from Tobago. At Grenada the ratio of deaths annually, per thousand of the mean strength of the troops, is not more than 6·6, while in St. Vincent's it is 10·5. *"Fort Charlotte is built on a very steep hill,* and about a mile and-a-half to the north west of Kingston." The Richmond Heights, though said to be more elevated, are immediately above St. George's. The quantity of finely powdered lime, which is constantly floating in the atmosphere of Barbados, is quite sufficient to account for pulmonary complaints in this island: but the ratio of annual deaths, which here amounts to 15·8 per thousand of the mean strength, is greatly increased by the number of invalids that are sent from the other islands for embarkation to England, and many of whom die before they can be embarked. St. Lucia, as was to be expected, has a ratio as high as 12·5. "The fort where the principal part of the troops are stationed, is built on the summit of a *very steep hill, about a mile and-a-half from Castries,"* the capital of the island. At Dominica the ratio is 8·3: for even here " the troops are principally quartered *on the*

summit of a table rock, overlooking the Town of Rosseau."
"This rock is surrounded by two deep and winding ravines, *one of which forms the bed of a mountain torrent,* the
other contains *many patches of moist and marshy ground.*"
Hence, we may believe, as is proved, that the mortality from fever, though not so great as at St. Lucia or
Trinidad, nor half of what takes place at Tobago, is
considerably above the average of the other Colonies.
But, as is well observed, " the most remarkable feature in
the mortality of the white troops in this island, is the
proportion of deaths by diseases of the bowels, which is
higher than by all the other diseases together 70·3 per
thousand of the mean strength.   Not having been in this
island I am unable to form any opinion as to the cause of
so great a mortality.   I cannot help thinking, however,
that there is some poisonous quality in the water which
the troops use, and not unlikely something that might
be remedied about the barrack privies.   " The troops at
Antigua are principally quartered *on a range of heights*
about 400 feet above the level of the sea, commanding
the entrance to English harbour." The dryness of the
atmosphere in this island is also remarkable : and, hence,
we find that the ratio of deaths from diseases of the lungs
is as high as nine per thousand.   At St. Kitt's " the
principal barracks are situated *on Brimstone Hill,* 700 *feet
above the level of the sea,*" and which " is precipitous on
every side, except where a narrow winding road forms an
approach to it from the beach ;" consequently, the deaths
here are as high as 9·5 per thousand.
     I have taken these numbers and remarks from the
Report before me, as they strongly corroborate the opi-

nion I have stated in this letter, and which I had formed
long before I left the West Indies. The next remarkable
circumstance which is proved by this Report is, the
greater mortality that prevails among the non-commissioned officers than even among the worst conducted of
the privates. This struck me so forcibly at Demerara
that I was at some pains to ascertain the cause; and I
sought for some explanation from the most intelligent of
these non-commissioned officers themselves. One respect-
able serjeant of the 25th regiment, who had served long
in the Colony, and was in the confidence of all his
brethren, gave me the following account:—he said " that,
although they had a mess of their own, and were enabled
by their higher pay to procure more fresh meat and better
vegetables than the men, still their craving for drink was
incessant. Their duties and their responsibility kept them
from mixing spirits with the water during the day, consequently the quantity of that element which they swallowed
(not always pure) tended greatly to injure their constitutions, and rendered them less able to bear up against acute
disease than the men who took spirits at all times;" but
the great and principal cause of their suffering arose from
a custom, which they had all found it necessary to adopt
and which, he said, was this : " when exhausted and worn
out with the duties and fatigues of the day, the time
arrived for their tumbling into bed, each took such a dose
of strong rum as was sufficient to make him dead drunk."
This was called "*putting on their night-cap*." It enabled
them to obtain some hours of sleep, or rather of quiet
rest, as it rendered them insensible to all the annoyances
of their barrack-rooms, and they got up in the morning

sufficiently refreshed and recruited for the next day's toil:
but when on guard this could not be done. " If such
duty returned only once or twice in the week it might be
borne with impunity; if oftener, or if for two or three
nights together, they were deprived of this (to them
invigorating) draught, they became so debilitated and
nervous that they were either carried off by *Delirium
tremens*, or fell a prey to the first attack of fever with
which they were affected." In fact, my Lord, their
physical powers had become too much depressed to
be easily restored to a healthy tone. That this was the
cause of the mortality in Demerara, I am quite certain :
and, I rather believe, the custom of taking a sleeping
dose of the same description was pretty general among
the non-commissioned officers throughout the command.

I quite agree with Captain Tulloch, that neither heat
nor moisture, nor the presence or absence of the trade
winds, are capable of themselves to produce any of those
sudden explosions of yellow fever which so frequently
and so fatally occur in our West India Colonies. But it
is their combination; and I have quite satisfied myself
that all the epidemic and endemical fevers of these Colonies, derive their origin from some subtle poison, called
into existence by that combination formed under some
special and peculiar influences, but the nature of which
still remains to be discovered. I am also convinced that
this poison is introduced into the system, *through the
medium of the stomach, and not of the lungs;* that it does
not consist in any vitiated quality of the air itself, but in
some poisonous matter which that air carries along with
it, and which, as is now proved, it will not elevate to a

greater height than 2500 feet above the level of the
sea. Yellow fever has never been known beyond that
height.

In my humble opinion, also, the nature or composition
of any soil has little effect in producing fever, in as far as
regards the superficial strata; but a great deal depends
upon the substratum. If a thin, or tolerably thin stratum
of comminuted earth or mould, is spread over a solid
rock, or an impervious substratum of clay, so that the
water or moisture which falls from the clouds, can only
penetrate to a moderate depth, and can never get beyond
the influence of the solar heat, then, my Lord, the
locality will always abound in what are called marsh
miasmata; and the harder and drier the surface becomes,
the more virulent will the poison be which is fetched up
from the stagnant water beneath. The mountain torrents
which originally had their courses over the naked rock,
or had hollowed them out of the accumulated beds of
argillaceous earth, are now generally filled up for a foot
or two in depth, with sand or small gravel. In the dry
season, these channels become apparently dry, and no
trace of water may appear for miles; still below the
surface, at a greater or less depth, according to the
continuance of the drought, and percolating through this
sand or gravel, there is a continued stream from which
the sun draws, or enables it to generate, that poison which
induces intermittent, remittent, or yellow fever. If,
however, the earth or substratum is porous, and to a
considerable depth, and beyond the reach of the surface
heat, then, whether the soil be wet or dry, a poor or a
rich mould, black, brown, or gray, the surface will be

healthy, and the marsh poison will only issue from the
margin of stagnant pools, or the banks of running streams.
Neither abundance of vegetable matter, nor its absence,
—neither the luxuriance of the growing mangrove, nor
the quantity of decaying vegetables,—have any great
effect in producing this secret assassin. So long as any
portion of the surface continues covered with water,
even in the worst marshes, that portion is free from
danger; and so it is with the mountain stream. The dis-
tillation then takes place only from their dried margins.
But when the pool or the river are entirely dried up,
there is an end of their insalubrity,—I mean in the deep
sandy or gravelly soils, as the depth to which that dryness
penetrates is too vast for the sun's influence to reach
beyond it.

I have partially analyzed the air from some of the
most pestilential marshes in British Guiana, and I found
it contained as much oxygen, and not more carbonic acid
gas, as that I had examined at Hampton Court; and the
azote seemed as pure. I found, however, a palpable
residuum, but whether of an animal or vegetable nature,
I had not time to determine. I had instituted a series
of experiments, and was pursuing them with great ardour,
when the caprice of a silly, passionate, old man, put an
end to them at an hour's notice. From the little I had
ascertained, and the few experiments I had made, on the
electrical conditions of the atmosphere, and the peculiar
influences that seemed to give a character to the prevailing
fevers, and other diseases, I had hoped to establish some
important results. But only one fact can I venture to
announce as fairly established, and it is this,—If a man's

face is perfectly covered with a veil of thin muslin, or silk gauze, and no air allowed to enter the mouth or nostrils, but what passes through that veil, he may sleep in the midst of the most pestilential marsh with perfect impunity, as regards intermittent fever. I had ascertained this, and had satisfied myself of its truth, before I was aware that it was no new discovery.

In choosing a military station, it matters little whether it is on the windward or leeward side of the island, on a level plain or on a high mountain. If the soil is such that the rain cannot penetrate beyond the sun's influence, it will always prove unhealthy, and the troops will be subject to fever. But there is one thing pretty certain, any insolated mountain in the neighbourhood of a pestilential marsh, will always be more unhealthy than the marsh itself. If there is a series of mountains, the summits of the first and second in the range, will be unhealthy, but the third will remain free from any appearance of fever. The building upon eminences, as was uniformly the case in the West Indies, from a belief that altitude gives security from the marsh poison, has been found a very fatal error in many instances. It proved no protection, as was soon discovered, against fever, and it has led to many other diseases, especially inflammation of the lungs, and perhaps also of the liver, which, as this report proves, have added not a little to that "great loss of life annually experienced in these colonies."

In all those stations where the permeable nature of the earth allows the rain-water to penetrate rapidly deep beneath the surface, a wet season will prove unhealthy, because the moisture cannot all escape the malignant in-

fluences that give origin to the poison, and more or less of
it, according to the quantity of rain that falls, will always
be generated,—whereas the quantity that falls in a dry
season, getting out of reach before it can be acted upon,
the station will always be healthy. But, on the contrary,
at a station where the soil is shallow, and the rock or im-
permeable clay-beds are very near to the surface, the
health of the troops will be the best when the season is
most wet, for then the soil being so supersaturated with
moisture, becomes as innocuous as the surface of the wide
spread lake. There will be no fever while the rains continue, but sad will be the fate of those that are doomed
to remain on the same spot when the dry weather has
commenced.

These remarks are offered as some explanation of the
hitherto rather paradoxical statements, which Captain
Tulloch has shown to be proved with respect to the
agency of marshes, and the physical and geological character of the soil. As regards the marsh-poison itself, and
the question so often asked, What is it? I can only,
like others, offer a conjecture, which is this: I consider
that, at particular seasons, or under peculiar influences,
certain living *essences* are called into existence, which
floating in the atmosphere, are swallowed in myriads,
and dissolving in the stomach, poison the vital fluids;
that, in proportion to the ravages committed upon these
fluids, we have the phenomena of fever more or less
developed. It has long been well-known that the first
symptom of the approach of intermittent fever, was the
altered condition of the blood, and in consequence the
vitiated quality of all the secretions from that fluid. We

know that the *ova* of insects will remain dormant in the earth, or in the water for years, and that not till some particular circumstances, or peculiar influences, call them into life, can their existence be known. We see millions of winged insects after, perhaps, a heavy shower, or a prolonged thunder-storm, burst all at once into existence, so as almost to darken the air. The clouds of sand-flies that stretch along the shores of British Guiana, and though individually scarcely perceptible, are so blood-thirsty and annoying as to surpass even the mosquito, are, I would say, a link in the chain which may connect the dragon-fly, (insect of the water also,) with the invisible but not less active insect that constitutes the *marsh miasmata.*

The qualities which my excellent friend Dr. Fergusson has noticed in his able and philosophical essay*, on the origin and history of this marsh poison, all tend to confirm my opinion. " It possesses," says he, "a singular attraction for the earth's surface, and umbrageous trees." " It creeps along the ground so as to concentrate and collect on the sides of the adjacent hills, and is certainly lost and absorbed by passing over a small surface of water." "The rarifying heat of the sun certainly dispels it, and it is only during the cooler temperature of the night, that it acquires body, concentration, and power." "All regular currents of wind have also the same effect." I may add, what is now also generally admitted, that it cannot rise in the atmosphere above a certain height; or rather, I would say, these invisible insects cannot live in so low a temperature as that which is found within the tropics, at an elevation of 2,500 feet above the level of the sea; and we

Edin. Philosoph. Transactions, 1820.

know, that even in England, when the temperature of the
air rises above a certain point, fever and ague were and
are always generated in our fenny counties. I question,
if a single mountain, rising out of a marshy plain, would
be quite free from the influence of the poison at even the
high elevation mentioned; but as regards a range of mountains, I know that the third from the marsh, as already
remarked, will prove quite healthy at a much lower elevation than that fixed upon by Humboldt, and even if it is
considerably lower than the two that intervene. The
more we penetrate into a mountainous country, the more
certain we are of finding a healthy locality within the
tropics ; and it is because, generally speaking, the islands
at the entrance of the Caribbean Sea, consist of a single
mountain only, with the soil that has accumulated at its
base, that they still are, and ever have been so very productive of remittent fevers. Jamaica alone, of all the
British Colonies, affords sufficient scope for finding a
healthy inland station ; though I am inclined to believe,
there are more than one sequestered spots within the
mountain range of Trinidad that the marsh-poison has
never reached, though not even so elevated as the barracks of Fort George, where as was soon discovered, no
white man could survive a week.

If in future it should ever become necessary to fix
upon a new station for our troops, or to select a fresh
locality for the erection of a barrack, the first duty of an
engineer will be to have the ground bored, so as to
ascertain the nature of the soil, and the depth of permeable strata. If sand, or gravel, prevail to the depth of
ten, fifteen, or still better, twenty feet, the station will be

healthy; but, if there are only two or three feet of these materials, and the subsoil is plastic clay, or solid rock, then, that locality is to be avoided. The salubrity of the sandy and gravelly soil, will also depend in some measure upon the facility of drainage, which the situation may admit of. If the water cannot be drawn freely from the depth to which it may have descended, it must accumulate and rise up towards the surface, and eventually, may become as pernicious as a more superficial moisture.

Whatever situation, therefore, is chosen, there should always be a sufficient fall to allow the water to be carried off from the lowest depth to which it can penetrate. I would refer to the remarks and returns from the stations of Fort Augusta, and Stoney Hill, in the Island of Jamaica; (the former, built at the extremity of a low neck of land, the latter, on a lofty eminence, 1300 feet above the level of the sea;) in corroboration of what is here recommended. The first is built upon a stratum *of sand covering a porous coral rock;* the last, on a flat top, between the ends of two high mountain ridges, and the soil is of a *reddish clay* mixed with sand. In the one, therefore, the water sinks beyond what I will call *fever depth;* in the other, it is retained and ready for action whenever a proper combination of other influences are brought into play.

Stoney Hill, it follows, as a matter of course, must be more subject to the ravages of epidemic fever than Fort Augusta; and, from Captain Tulloch's Tables, we find that it is so in the proportion of $70\frac{1}{2}$, $55\frac{1}{2}$, per thousand. And even as regards diseases of the lungs, I hold that these two stations tend to confirm, rather than refute, my theory, as to the principal causes of such complaints. Fort Augusta, be it remembered, though situated on a level plain, is placed between the towns of Kingston and Port Royal, and not more than four miles from either; consequently, we may suppose the soldiers will frequently have leave to visit both places, and lingering, as they always will do, in the grog-shops, until the very last moment has expired, they start off at a run, and are obliged to keep it up that they may reach the garrison before the roll call.

Now, my Lord, a long race on a level plain, is just as dangerous as a shorter one up a steep ascent, and the soldier when he arrives at Fort Augusta from Port Royal, or Kingston, is as exhausted and excited as he would be in climbing from Scarburrough to Fort King George in Tobago; and the cool sea breezes are just as likely to check perspiration as any other cool breeze. Stoney Hill, on the contrary, though situated on an eminence, has no town at its base; the men have no temptation to wander down the hill, or to hasten up it; the can-teens are on the flat top of the hill, and within the com-pass of the twenty acres which are occupied by the parade and barrack buildings; and, although from the locality, I would look for a considerable number of cases of acute catarrh, I certainly should not expect anything like the same average number of fatal cases of inflam-mation of the lungs,—the great exciting cause being entirely wanting.

In conclusion, I have only one word more with regard to elevation. No matter how high you pitch your tent, if under the range of 2500 feet, and if the hill is nearest to the plain or marsh, (that is the front in the range,) you will never escape the ravages of the fever poison. And the higher you ascend, the more virulent will it become, *if there is a still higher peak,* of the same range adjoining your locality. Even that higher peak will be unhealthy; *but the next beyond it, whether higher or lower, will be free from all danger.*

I have the honour to be,

My Lord,

Your very faithful servant,

ANDREW HALLIDAY,

Deputy Inspector-General of Army Hospitals.

HUNTINGDON LODGE, DUMFRIES,
March 8th, 1839.

Printed in the United States
By Bookmasters